I have compiled this work to be of benefit to all people, I have made an effort to provide this information, and I do not claim any copyrights.

With all love

SeventyEight

Table of Contents

1. Understanding Aging
1.1 The Aging Process
1.2 Common Aging-Related Conditions

2. Nutrition and Hydration
2.1 Nutritional Needs of the Elderly
2.2 Hydration Importance

3. Physical Health and Activity
3.1 Importance of Regular Exercise
3.2 Preventing Injuries and Falls

4. Medication Management
4.1 Understanding Medications
4.2 Organizing Medications

5. Emotional and Social Well-being
5.1 Supporting Mental Health
5.2 Coping with Grief and Loss

6. Caregiver Support
6.1 Recognizing Caregiver Challenges
6.2 Resources for Caregivers

7. Conclusion

1. Understanding Aging

1.1 The Aging Process

Aging is a multifaceted, natural process characterized by a series of complex physical, cognitive, and emotional changes. Understanding these changes is crucial for providing effective care and ensuring the dignity and well-being of elderly individuals.

Definition:

Aging involves progressive physiological changes that lead to physical and mental decline over time, affecting overall health and quality of life.

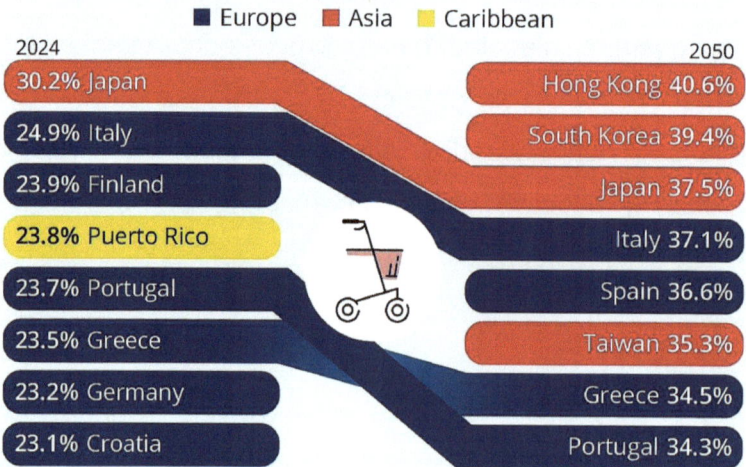

Dataset

Rank	Oldest Populations 2024	Rank	Oldest Populations 2050
1	Japan	1	Hong Kong
2	Italy	2	South Korea
3	Finland	3	Japan
4	Puerto Rico	4	Italy
5	Portugal	5	Spain
6	Greece	6	Taiwan
7	Germany	7	Greece
8	Croatia	8	Portugal

Data sources

https://www.statista.com/chart/29345/countries-and-territories-with-the-highest-share-of-people-aged-65-and-older/

https://www.un.org/development/desa/dspd/wp-content/uploads/sites/22/2023/01/2023wsr-fullreport.pdf

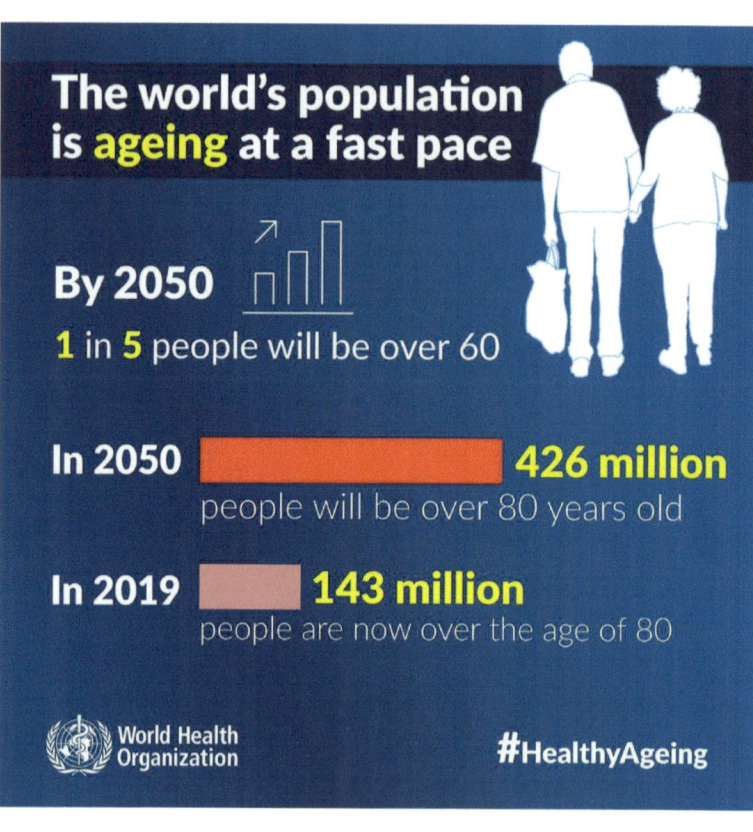

Physical Changes:

Aging affects mobility, sensory perception, and organ function. As muscle mass decreases and bone density declines, elderly individuals may experience reduced strength and balance. Caregivers must adapt living environments by installing safety features, such as grab bars, improving lighting, and removing tripping hazards, to enhance mobility and minimize the risk of falls.

Cognitive Changes:

Cognitive decline, including conditions like dementia and Alzheimer's disease, is a significant concern. Caregivers should foster a cognitively stimulating environment by incorporating memory-enhancing activities, such as puzzles, reading, and engaging in social interactions. These activities can help slow cognitive deterioration and promote brain health. Early diagnosis of cognitive issues is vital, allowing for better planning and access to appropriate treatments, ultimately enabling individuals to maintain a higher quality of life.

Emotional and Psychological Aspects:

Elderly individuals may experience loneliness, depression, or anxiety due to lifestyle changes, loss of independence, and social isolation. It is crucial to maintain regular social interactions through family visits, community programs, and technology solutions like video calls to keep elderly individuals connected with their loved ones. Mental health support, including counseling and therapy, should be sought when necessary.

Biological Changes:

Cellular Aging:

Aging at the cellular level occurs due to genetic factors and environmental influences, such as exposure to toxins. Mitigating cellular aging through proper nutrition, regular exercise, and stress management can improve longevity and health.

Organ Function:

With age, organ function naturally deteriorates, increasing vulnerability to various health issues. Proactive medical care, including regular check-ups and early intervention strategies, such as rehabilitation and lifestyle modifications, can help maintain quality of life and functional independence.

Metabolism:

Aging slows metabolic processes, necessitating dietary adjustments to prevent weight gain and nutrient deficiencies. A balanced diet, rich in vitamins and minerals, tailored to meet the changing needs of the body, is essential.

Psychological Aspects:

Coping with Loss:

Aging often comes with significant loss, such as the passing of loved ones, which can lead to grief and emotional distress. Building emotional resilience through support groups, counseling, and fostering strong social connections can help elderly individuals navigate these challenges.

Loneliness:

Loneliness can significantly impact mental health in older adults. Technology solutions, such as video calls and social media, can help elderly individuals maintain relationships with distant family and friends, reducing feelings of isolation.

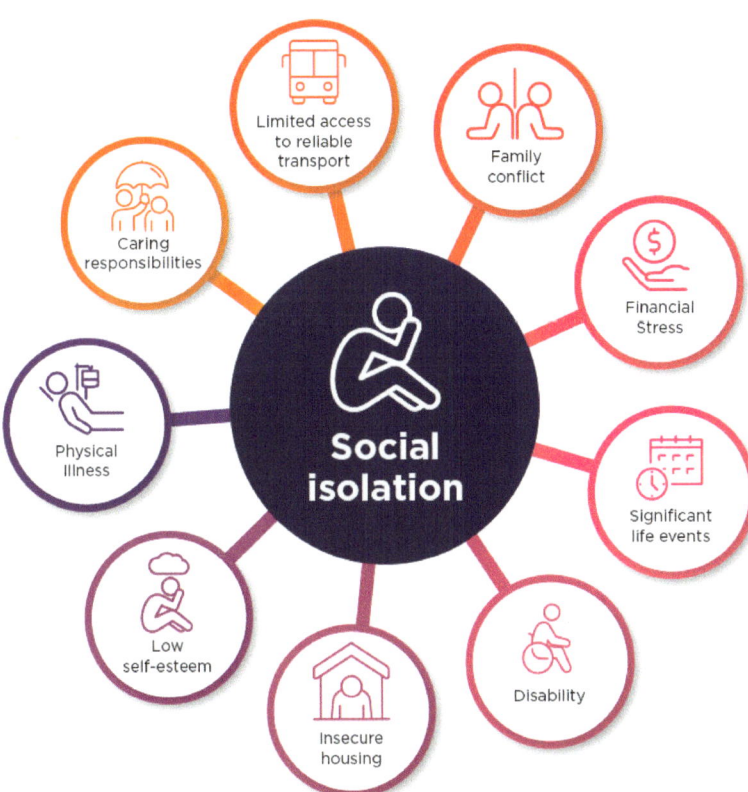

Social Implications:

Changing Roles:
Retirement and health challenges may limit elderly individuals' roles in society, leading to a sense of loss of purpose. Programs focused on lifelong learning, volunteer opportunities, and mentorship can help preserve their sense of identity and contribution to the community.

1.2 Common Aging-Related Conditions

Chronic Illnesses:
As people age, they are more likely to develop chronic health conditions such as arthritis, diabetes, and heart disease. These conditions can significantly impact quality of life, but early detection and intervention, along with lifestyle changes, can improve outcomes. Managing these illnesses through regular medical check-ups, adhering to prescribed treatments, maintaining physical activity, and

adopting a healthy diet can help prevent complications and promote better overall health.

1. Arthritis:
Definition:
A group of conditions that cause inflammation and stiffness in the joints, leading to pain and reduced mobility.
Causes:
Aging, genetics, joint injuries, and obesity can contribute to the development of arthritis.
Prevention:
Regular physical activity, maintaining a healthy weight, and avoiding overuse of joints are critical in reducing the risk.
Solution:
Treatment options include medications for pain relief and inflammation, physical therapy to improve joint function, and, in severe cases, surgical interventions such as joint replacement.

2. Diabetes:

Definition:

A metabolic disorder characterized by the body's inability to effectively regulate blood sugar levels, leading to elevated glucose levels in the blood.

Causes:

Risk factors include genetics, poor diet, physical inactivity, and obesity.

Prevention:

Healthy eating, regular exercise, and maintaining a healthy weight can help reduce the risk of developing diabetes.

Solution:

Management often includes medication (including insulin for type 1 diabetes), lifestyle modifications, and regular monitoring of blood sugar levels to prevent complications.

3. Heart Disease:

Definition:

A range of cardiovascular conditions affecting the heart's ability to function properly, including coronary artery disease and heart failure.

Causes:

Poor diet, sedentary lifestyle, smoking, and high cholesterol contribute to heart disease.

Prevention:

A heart-healthy diet rich in fruits, vegetables, whole grains, and lean proteins, along with regular exercise and smoking cessation, can significantly lower risk.

Solution:

Management may involve medications to control blood pressure and cholesterol levels, lifestyle changes, and, in some cases, surgical procedures.

Cognitive Decline:

Cognitive conditions such as dementia and Alzheimer's disease are significant concerns for older adults, affecting memory, decision-making, and overall daily functioning. Engaging in mentally stimulating activities, including puzzles, reading, and participating in social interactions, can help slow down cognitive decline. Early diagnosis plays a crucial role in enabling better planning and treatment options, providing individuals with improved strategies to manage the condition and maintain their quality of life.

1. Dementia:

Definition:

A general term for a decline in cognitive ability severe enough to interfere with daily life, affecting memory, thinking, and social abilities.

Causes:

Risk factors include age, genetics, and lifestyle factors like smoking and poor diet.

Prevention:

Engaging in mentally stimulating activities, maintaining a healthy diet, and participating in regular physical activity can help reduce the risk of dementia.

Solution:

Treatment may include medications to manage symptoms, cognitive therapy to enhance function, and support programs to assist caregivers and individuals.

2. Alzheimer's Disease:
Definition:

A progressive neurological disorder and the most common cause of dementia, characterized by memory loss and cognitive decline.

Causes:

Genetic predisposition, age, and environmental factors contribute to its development.

Prevention:

Healthy lifestyle choices, including a balanced diet and regular exercise, may help reduce the risk of Alzheimer's disease.

Solution:

Management strategies include medications to temporarily improve symptoms, cognitive exercises to enhance brain function, and caregiver support to facilitate daily living.

Mental Health Issues:

Depression and anxiety are prevalent among the elderly and often go untreated, yet addressing these challenges is essential for their emotional well-being and overall quality of life. A combination of therapy, medication, and strong social support can effectively manage these mental health issues, helping older adults maintain a positive outlook and improve their day-to-day functioning.

1. Depression:

Definition:

A mood disorder characterized by persistent feelings of sadness and loss of interest in life, affecting daily functioning.

Causes:

Factors contributing to depression include life changes, the loss of loved ones, chronic illness, and social isolation.

Prevention:

Encouraging regular social interactions, physical activity, and creating a supportive home environment can significantly reduce the risk of depression.

Solution:

Effective treatment may involve therapy (such as cognitive-behavioral therapy), medication, and participation in support groups to foster community connections.

2. Anxiety:

Definition:

A mental health condition marked by excessive worry, fear, or nervousness that interferes with daily activities.

Causes:

Common triggers include health issues, changes in living situations, and feelings of loneliness.

Prevention:

Regular participation in social and physical activities, mindfulness practices, and stress reduction techniques can help alleviate anxiety symptoms.

Solution:

Management may involve cognitive-behavioral therapy (CBT) and medications such as anti-anxiety prescriptions, providing effective coping strategies and emotional support.

10 Common Chronic Conditions for Adults 65+

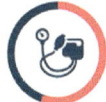
Hypertension (High Blood Pressure)
60%

High Cholesterol
51%

Obesity
42%

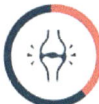
Arthritis
35%

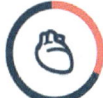
Ischemic / Coronary Heart Disease
29%

Diabetes
27%

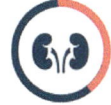

Chronic Kidney Disease
25%

Heart Failure
15%

Depression
16%

Alzheimer's Disease and Dementia
12%

Source: Centers for Medicare & Medicaid Services, Chronic Conditions Prevalence State/County Table: All Fee-for-Service Beneficiaries. Centers for Disease Control and Prevention. Adult Obesity Facts.

© 2024 National Council on Aging All Rights Reserved

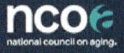

Percentage of Older Adults with Chronic Conditions	
High cholesterol	58.2
Hypertension	56.7
Arthritis	48.7
Cancer	23.1
Diabetes	20.5
Heart disease	17.9
Ulcers	11.3
Stroke	7.2
Asthma	6.9
Kidney disease	5.1
Chronic bronchitis	5.0
Emphysema	4.0

Adapted from CDC National Health Interview 2014

2. Nutrition and Hydration

2.1 Nutritional Needs of the Elderly

Proper nutrition is paramount for maintaining health and preventing age-related diseases among elderly individuals. A balanced diet that emphasizes a variety of fruits, vegetables, lean proteins, healthy fats, and whole grains is essential for promoting longevity and overall well-being. As metabolism naturally slows with age, the elderly have specific nutritional requirements to help maintain health and quality of life. Here are the key nutrients essential for elderly individuals:

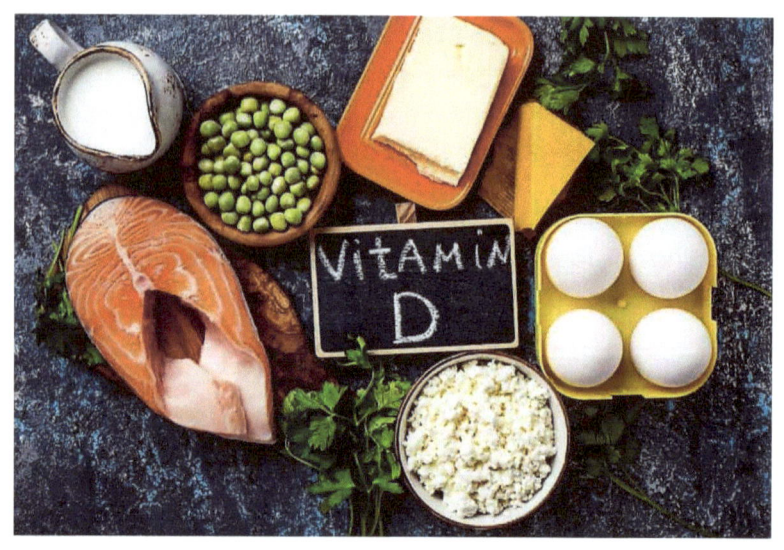
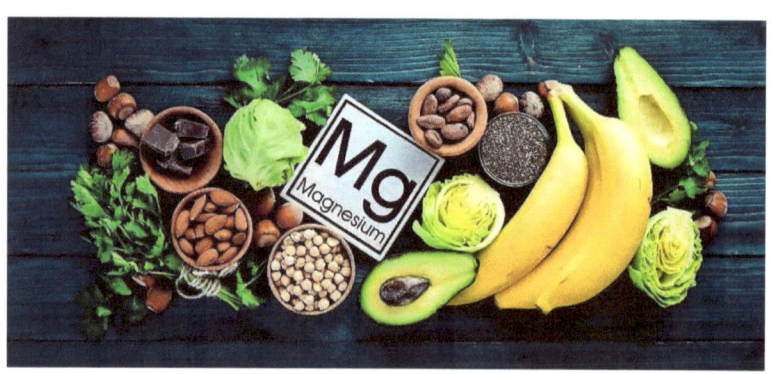

TOP NUTRITION TIPS FOR AGING WELL

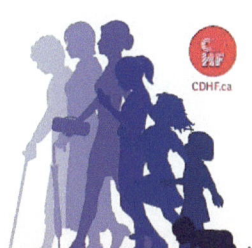

When it comes to diet QUALITY over QUANTITY

With lifestyle changes that come with transition to older adulthood, nutrition needs may be different at this stage.

Key dietary elements that are important to keep up with as you age include:

Vitamin B12 is responsible for red blood cell formation, cellular metabolism, nerve/cognitive functioning, bone health, and more.

Treatment may include:
- B12 intramuscular injections
- Supplements
- Increase B12-rich sources of food

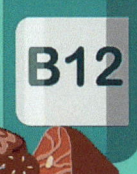

Vitamin B12 rich foods:

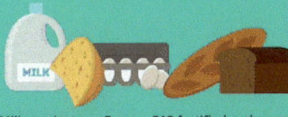

Milk products | Eggs | B12-fortified grain products | Soy products | Seafood | A variety of meats

*Aim for 2.4 mcg daily for men and women.

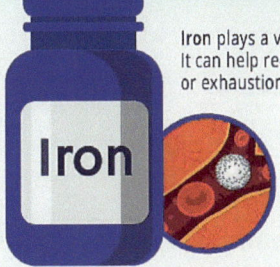

Iron plays a vital role in blood production. It can help reduce feelings of tiredness or exhaustion.

Treatment may include:
- An iron-rich diet
- Use of prescribed iron pills

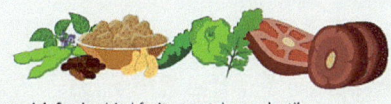

Iron-rich foods: dried fruits, meat, beans, lentils, iron-fortified cereals, and dark leafy green vegetables.

* The recommended iron for seniors is 8 mg daily for both men and women (post-menopausal).

1. Proteins:

Function:

Vital for maintaining muscle mass and repairing tissues.

Sources:

Lean meats, beans, eggs, fish, and legumes.

Importance for the Elderly:

Sufficient protein intake is crucial to combat muscle loss (sarcopenia) and weakness, which can impair mobility and independence.

2. Fats:

Function:

Provides a concentrated source of energy and supports cell function.

Sources:

Healthy fats such as olive oil, avocados, nuts, and fatty fish.

Importance for the Elderly:

Unsaturated fats help reduce inflammation and support heart health, essential for preventing cardiovascular diseases.

3. Fiber:

Function:

Promotes healthy digestion and prevents constipation.

Sources:

Whole grains, fruits, vegetables, and legumes.

Importance for the Elderly:

A high-fiber diet reduces the risk of digestive issues and helps regulate blood sugar levels, which is particularly important for managing diabetes.

4. Water (Hydration):

Function:

Vital for all bodily functions, including digestion, nutrient absorption, and temperature regulation.

Sources:

Water, herbal teas, soups, and fruits/vegetables with high water content.

Importance for the Elderly:

Prevents dehydration, a common issue due to decreased thirst perception in older adults.

5. Calcium:

Function:

Essential for maintaining strong bones and preventing osteoporosis.

Sources:

Dairy products, fortified plant-based milks, and leafy greens.

Importance for the Elderly:

Adequate calcium intake prevents fractures and supports overall bone density.

6. Omega-3 Fatty Acids:

Function:

Supports brain health, reduces inflammation, and promotes cardiovascular health.

Sources:

Fatty fish like salmon, flaxseeds, walnuts, and chia seeds.

Importance for the Elderly:

Omega-3s can help reduce cognitive decline and maintain cardiovascular health, vital for longevity.

While these nutrients are crucial for elderly individuals, barriers such as difficulty in meal preparation, reduced appetite, and economic constraints may hinder proper nutrition. Caregivers play a critical role in assisting with meal planning, shopping, and cooking to ensure access to a wide variety of nutritious foods.

2.2 Hydration Importance

Signs of Dehydration:

Dehydration can significantly impact the health and well-being of older adults, leading to serious complications. Common signs include:

- Dry mouth and decreased saliva production
- Fatigue and lethargy
- Dizziness or lightheadedness
- Confusion and cognitive changes
- Reduced urine output and darker urine, indicating concentrated waste products due to insufficient fluid intake

Important to note :

Cognitive decline and an increased risk of falls can result from dehydration, affecting concentration and coordination. Older adults often do not feel thirst as acutely as younger individuals due to age-related changes in the body's thirst mechanism and certain medications that may reduce the sensation of thirst. This makes regular hydration even more crucial.

Encouraging Fluid Intake:

To promote adequate hydration, caregivers should encourage regular fluid intake throughout the day. Strategies include:
- Offering water frequently and integrating hydration into daily routines.
- Making fluids readily available, using flavored waters, herbal teas, and broth-based soups to enhance appeal.
- Incorporating fruits and vegetables with high water content, such as cucumbers, watermelon, oranges, and celery, into meals and snacks.

- Setting reminders or using hydration tracking apps can help older adults remember to drink fluids regularly. Creating a pleasant environment for hydration—such as enjoying tea time or serving meals that include soups or stews—can encourage fluid consumption in a social setting.
- Regularly assessing hydration status and adjusting fluid intake based on activity levels, weather conditions, and individual health needs will further ensure optimal hydration for older adults.

By fostering an environment that prioritizes nutrition and hydration, caregivers can significantly enhance the quality of life for the elderly, helping them maintain independence and vitality.

3. Physical Health and Activity

3.1 Importance of Regular Exercise

Regular physical activity is essential for enhancing the quality of life among older adults. It not only significantly reduces the risk of chronic diseases such as heart disease, diabetes, and obesity, but it also plays a crucial role in improving mental health by alleviating symptoms of depression and anxiety. Furthermore, engaging in regular exercise helps maintain independence, allowing seniors to perform daily activities without assistance. Incorporating low-impact exercises into their routines—such as walking, swimming, and strength training—is vital for preserving mobility, flexibility, and overall physical strength.

Types of Suitable Exercises:

1. Strength Training:

Purpose:
Essential for building muscle mass and bone density.

Methods:
Utilizing resistance bands, free weights, or body-weight exercises.

Importance for the Elderly:
As individuals age, they naturally experience muscle loss, known as sarcopenia, which can lead to frailty and decreased mobility. Engaging in strength training at least twice a week helps improve muscle strength, enhance functional capacity, and reduce the risk of osteoporosis and fractures.

2. Flexibility Exercises:

Purpose:

Improve mobility and prevent stiffness.

Methods:

Stretching, yoga, and gentle movements that promote flexibility.

Importance for the Elderly:

These exercises help maintain a healthy range of motion in joints, reducing the risk of injuries. Regular flexibility training enhances posture, balance, and overall body awareness—key factors for daily activities and fall prevention.

3. Low-Impact Cardio:

Purpose:

Enhance cardiovascular health without stressing the joints.

Methods:

Walking, cycling, swimming, and other moderate-intensity aerobic activities.

Importance for the Elderly:

Engaging in at least 150 minutes of moderate-intensity aerobic activity each week can improve heart health, increase stamina, and promote better circulation. Additionally, low-impact cardio exercises contribute to weight management and improve mood through the release of endorphins.

3.2 Preventing Injuries and Falls

Preventing injuries and falls is critical in elderly care, as falls are a leading cause of serious injury among older adults. Caregivers can implement specific strategies to significantly reduce the risk of falls, thereby enhancing the safety and well-being of seniors.

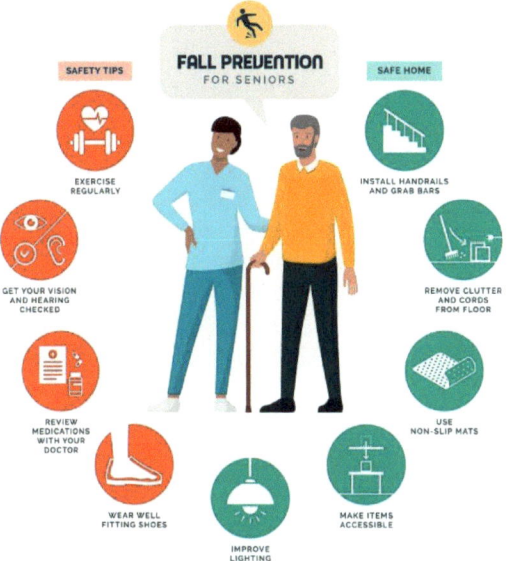

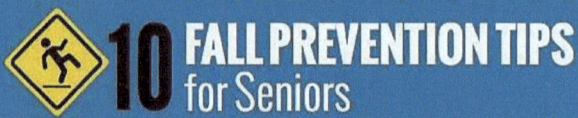

10 FALL PREVENTION TIPS for Seniors

June is National Safety Awareness Month — The National Safety Council has designated the third week of the month – the week of June 20th – to raise awareness around falls and fall prevention.

Falls remain a leading cause for injury in the United States: in fact, one in three older adults falls each year. In 2013 alone, over 2.5 million non-fatal falls were treated in the emergency room. Although falls may be more common in older adults, they can happen to anyone of any age, and there are many things you can do both in and out of the home to decrease the risk of falling.

Below are 10 Simple Tips for Fall Prevention from the National Safety Council and Other Resources

1. **Remove tripping hazards** such as books and papers, shoes, and boxes from stairs and hallways, and secure rugs.[1]

2. **Install grab-bars** in the bathroom, both around the toilet and in the shower.[1]

3. Keep frequently used items within **easy reach**, so you don't have to climb or strain for them.[1]

4. Make sure that both inside and outside the home has **adequate lighting** so you can see your path while walking.[1]

5. **Check and repair** any damages to walkways or steps regularly.[1]

6. **Wear sensible shoes** with nonskid soles and a proper fit.[2]

7. Poor vision is a major factor in falls. **Get an eye exam** at least once a year to keep prescriptions current and eyes functioning their best.[3]

8. Consider adding extra personal security by using a **mobile alert systems with GPS** to access emergency help at any time.

9. **Medication errors** are one of the main catalysts for falls. Keep an updated medication list, as well as all current labels attached to the bottle. Make sure to take the instructed dose, and talk to the pharmacist about any questions.[4]

10. **Stay active!** Even gentle exercise can increase strength and balance, helping to reduce the risk of falls.[5,6]

---

[1] http://www.nsc.org/NSCDocuments_Advocacy/Fact%20Sheets/Slips-Trips-and-Falls.pdf
[2] http://www.mayoclinic.org/healthy-lifestyle/healthy-aging/in-depth/fall-prevention/art-20047358
[3] http://www.healio.com/optometry/primary-care-optometry/news/print/primary-care-optometry-news/%7B9705b63b-ca71-4c57-b838-59e9e764e190%7D/optometrists-can-play-significant-role-in-fall-prevention-for-older-adults
[4] http://www.aplaceformom.com/blog/1-27-2014-medication-management-tips
[5] http://www.nsc.org/learn/safety-knowledge/Pages/safety-at-home-falls.aspx
[6] http://www.mayoclinic.org/healthy-lifestyle/healthy-aging/in-depth/fall-prevention/art-20047358

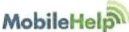

Home Safety Modifications:

Assess the Home Environment:
Identifying potential hazards is crucial for fall prevention.

Common Modifications:
- Improve lighting, especially in stairways and hallways, to enhance visibility.
- Install grab bars in bathrooms to provide support.
- Secure rugs to prevent slipping and remove clutter from walking paths to create a safer living space.
- Ensure that furniture is stable and frequently used items are within easy reach to minimize risks.

Balance and Strength Training:
Focus on Balance and Strength: Exercises that enhance balance and strength are particularly effective in reducing fall risk.

Recommended Activities:

Incorporate tai chi, balance-focused yoga, and targeted strength training exercises that improve stability and coordination.

Benefits: These exercises strengthen the lower body and enhance proprioception, which is the body's ability to sense its position in space. By incorporating balance training into regular exercise routines, older adults can navigate their environments more confidently, significantly reducing the likelihood of fall-related injuries.

Incorporating regular physical activity and safety measures into the daily routines of older adults is essential for promoting long-term health, independence, and overall well-being. Caregivers play a vital role in facilitating these activities and modifications, helping seniors maintain an active and safe lifestyle.

4. Medication Management

4.1 Understanding Medications

As individuals age, they often require multiple medications to manage various health conditions, leading to a phenomenon known as polypharmacy. This refers to the concurrent use of several drugs, which can increase the risk of adverse drug interactions, side effects, and health complications. It is essential for caregivers and healthcare providers to regularly review the medication regimens of elderly individuals, ensuring that each medication is necessary, effective, and safe. This review process helps identify potential drug interactions and allows for the elimination of unnecessary medications that may contribute to confusion or health deterioration.

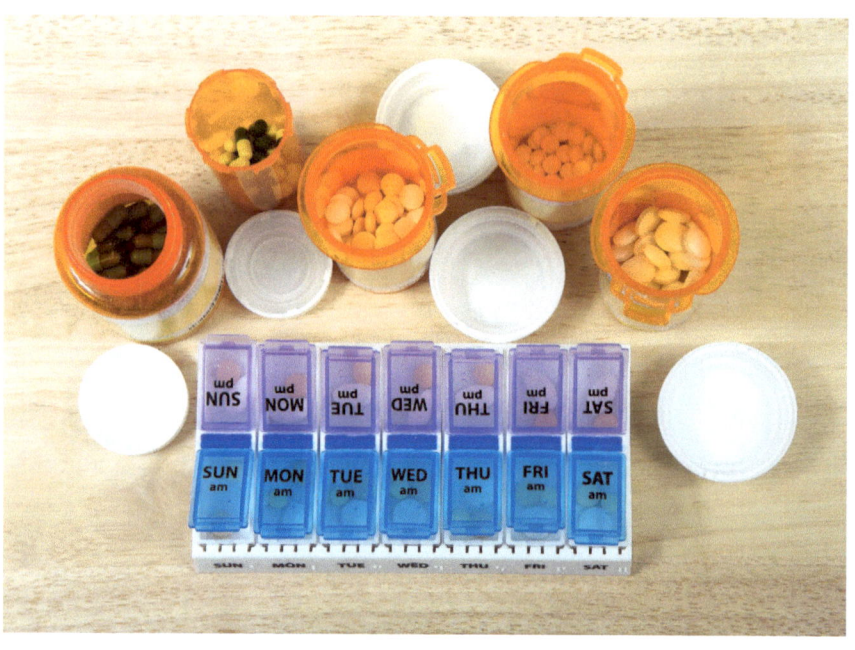

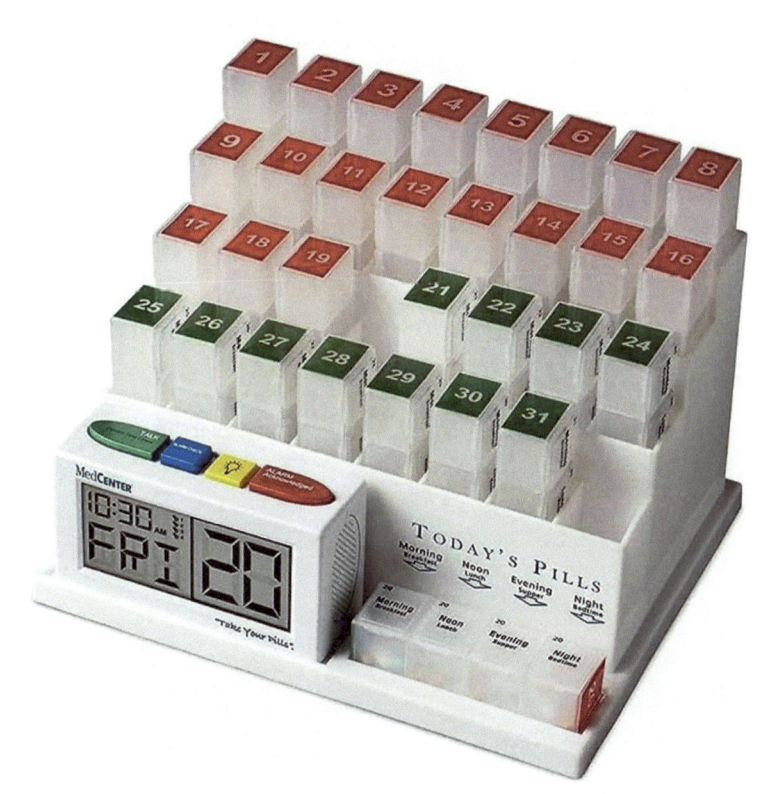

Common Medications:

Older adults may be prescribed a range of medications, including:

- Antihypertensives: For managing high blood pressure.

- Anticoagulants: To prevent blood clots.

- Antidepressants: For mental health support.

- Diabetes Medications: To help regulate blood sugar levels.

Understanding the purpose and effects of each medication is crucial for achieving optimal health outcomes.

Adherence: Non-adherence to medication regimens is a prevalent issue among the elderly, often caused by factors such as forgetfulness, confusion, or complex dosing schedules. To enhance adherence, caregivers can implement several strategies, including:

- Simplifying Medication Schedules: Streamlining dosing times can make it easier to remember.

- Providing Clear Instructions: Ensuring that instructions are easy to understand and follow.

- Using Pill Organizers: Categorizing medications by day or time can help individuals keep track of their dosages.

Establishing a routine for taking medications, along with regular check-ins to remind individuals about their regimens, can significantly improve adherence and health outcomes.

4.2 Organizing Medications

Tools for Management:

Effective medication management is critical to ensuring that elderly individuals take their medications as prescribed. Various tools can simplify this process, making it easier for both seniors and their caregivers:

- **Digital Reminders:** Smartphone apps or automated text alerts can prompt individuals to take their medications at the right times.

- **Automated Pill Dispensers:** These devices dispense the correct dosages at scheduled times, reducing the risk of missed or incorrect doses.

- **Visual Aids:** Using medication charts or color-coded labels can help elderly individuals and caregivers track medications effectively. These aids serve as quick references that simplify understanding when and how to take medications. Caregivers should maintain up-to-date lists of all medications, including dosages and prescribing physicians, for easy reference during medical appointments. This practice not only ensures better coordination among healthcare providers but also empowers elderly individuals to actively participate in their medication management, contributing to improved health outcomes.

By implementing structured medication management strategies, caregivers can enhance the effectiveness of treatment plans, reduce the risk of adverse effects, and improve the overall health and well-being of elderly individuals.

5. Emotional and Social Well-being

5.1 Supporting Mental Health

Combating Loneliness:

Loneliness is a significant concern for many elderly individuals, often leading to feelings of sadness and depression. To combat loneliness, it is essential to encourage participation in community events, social programs, and clubs tailored for older adults. These gatherings not only provide opportunities for social interaction but also foster a sense of belonging and community. Regular communication with family and friends—whether through phone calls, video chats, or in-person visits—is also crucial for emotional well-being. Caregivers can facilitate these connections by organizing family gatherings, setting up technology for virtual meetings, or planning outings that allow seniors to engage with their loved ones.

Engaging in Activities:

Active engagement in various activities is vital for maintaining mental health. Social games, such as bingo or card games, promote interaction and can enhance cognitive function while providing entertainment. Group activities—such as exercise classes, art workshops, or book clubs—encourage socialization and create a sense of camaraderie among participants. Additionally, hobbies like gardening, crafting, or cooking offer creative outlets and opportunities for social engagement when shared with others. These activities can significantly improve mental health and reduce feelings of isolation, promoting overall well-being.

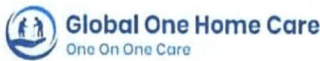

Sample Daily Schedule for Elderly

Use this sample schedule to create the most appropriate routine for your elderly loved one. You can pick any given activity at the time, from the list of activities.

Time	Activity	Details
Morning		
7:00am to 8:00am	Wake-Up Routine	Wake-Up, Morning Hygiene (brushing teeth, washing face, bathing), Morning medication
8:00am to 9:00am	Breakfast	Nutritious meal tailored to dietary needs (vegetarian, carnivore, balanced diet)
9:00am to 10:30am	Morning activities	Light Exercise (stretching, bed exercises, living room exercises), Outdoor Activities (gardening, park walks, pet care)
10:30am to 12:00pm	Mental Stimulation	Puzzles, reading, book clubs
Afternoon		
12:00pm to 12:30pm	Lunch	Balanced and nutritious meal (vegetarian, carnivore, balanced diet)
12:30pm to 1:00pm	Hydration	Encouraging fluid intake (water, herbal teas, diluted juices)
1:00pm to 2:30pm	Social Interaction	Visiting friends, community events, playing games
2:30pm to 3:30pm	Rest Time	Nap time, quiet time with calming music or meditative practices

Evening			
5:30pm to 6:00pm	Dinner		Nutritional and easy to digest meal (vegetarian, carnivore, balanced diet)
6:00pm	Evening Medication		Organize medications using a pill organizer
6:30pm to 8:30pm	Relaxation Activities		Watching TV, listening to music, light reading.
Night			
8:30pm to 9:00 pm	Night Hygiene		Brushing teeth, washing face, changing into nightwear, Consistent bedtime routine, ensuring comfortable bedding, temperature control, safety measures (night lights)
9:00 pm to 9:30 pm	Bedtime Routine		Consistent bedtime routine, ensuring comfortable bedding, temperature control, safety measures (night lights)

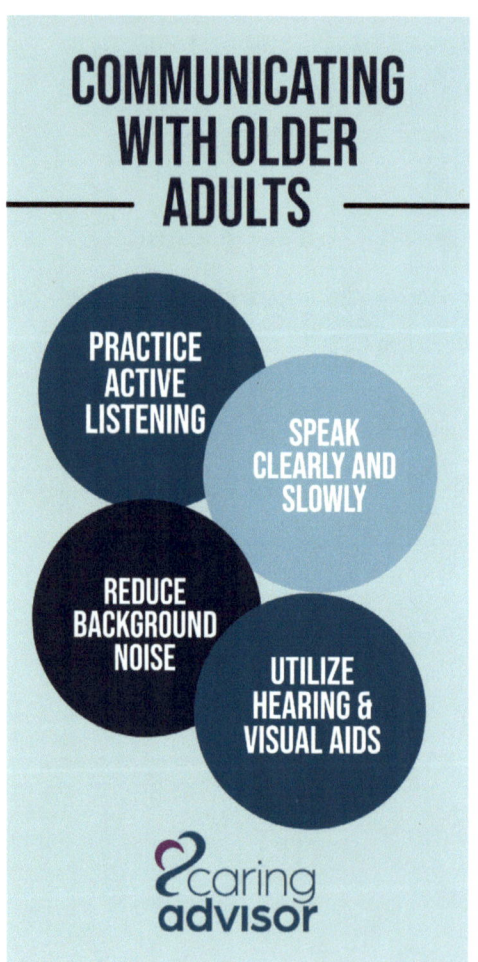

5.2 Coping with Grief and Loss

Grief Management:
Coping with grief and loss can be particularly challenging for older adults, who may have already experienced the loss of friends, family members, or partners. Providing access to counseling, therapy, and support groups that specialize in grief management is crucial. These resources offer elderly individuals a safe space to express their feelings, share their experiences, and learn coping strategies. Professional therapists can guide individuals through the grieving process, helping them navigate their emotions and avoid prolonged periods of depression.

Support groups—whether in-person or online—can foster a sense of community among those experiencing similar losses, allowing individuals to connect, share stories, and support one another. Encouraging participation in these support systems can help elderly individuals process their grief healthily, promoting emotional healing and resilience. By addressing grief constructively, caregivers can help seniors maintain their emotional health, fostering a sense of hope and the ability to move forward after loss.

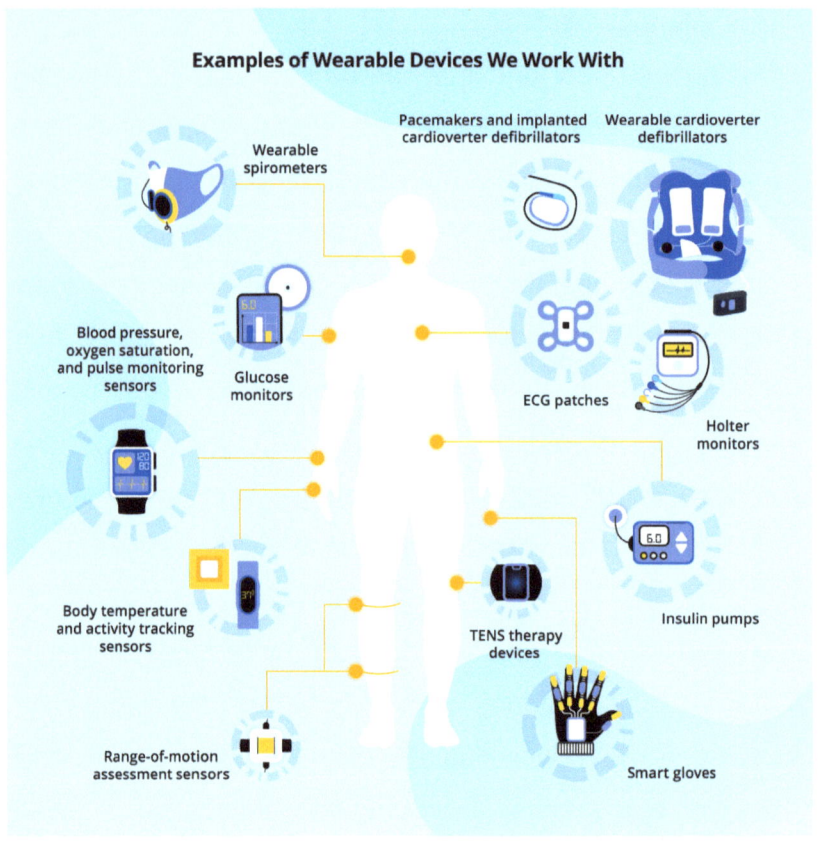

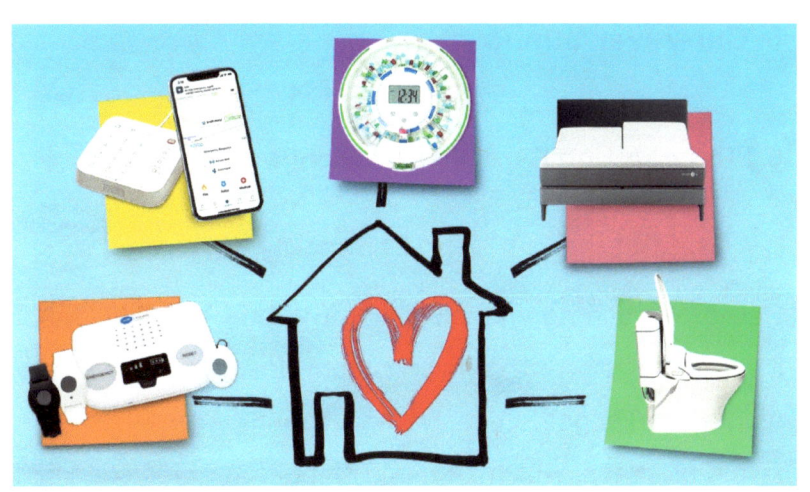

6. Caregiver Support

6.1 Recognizing Caregiver Challenges

Caregiver Burnout:
Caregiving can be an incredibly rewarding experience, but it often comes with significant physical, emotional, and mental challenges. Caregivers frequently experience high levels of stress, which can lead to burnout. This condition is characterized by fatigue, emotional exhaustion, irritability, and feelings of being overwhelmed. Recognizing the signs of caregiver burnout early is crucial, as it can impact not only the caregiver's well-being but also the quality of care provided to the elderly individual. Regular assessments of one's emotional and physical state can help caregivers identify when they are reaching their limits. Symptoms such as difficulty sleeping, withdrawal from social activities, and increased anxiety are indicators that a caregiver may need support.

Prevention Strategies:

Preventing caregiver burnout requires proactive strategies. Taking regular breaks is essential for maintaining mental health; even short periods away from caregiving duties can help recharge emotional batteries. Caregivers can also benefit from joining support groups, where they can share experiences, gain insights, and receive encouragement from others in similar situations. Respite care services, which provide professional caregivers for short periods, can be a valuable resource. These services allow primary caregivers the time they need to rest, attend to personal matters, or simply take a moment for themselves, ultimately enhancing their ability to provide compassionate care.

6.2 Resources for Caregivers

Access to Support Services:

Caregivers should have access to various resources designed to enhance their skills and provide necessary support. Training programs focusing on caregiving techniques—such as effective communication, managing medications, and understanding age-related health issues—can empower caregivers with knowledge and confidence. Additionally, mental health support is critical; counseling services tailored for caregivers can address the unique stressors they face, offering coping strategies and emotional relief.

Community Resources:

Community organizations often provide valuable resources for caregivers, including workshops, educational seminars, and networking opportunities. These programs can cover topics such as time management, stress reduction techniques, and self-care strategies, equipping caregivers with the tools they need to handle their responsibilities effectively. Furthermore, local resources like meal delivery services, transportation assistance, and in-home care agencies can alleviate some of the burdens associated with caregiving, allowing caregivers to focus on the emotional and relational aspects of their role. By connecting with these resources, caregivers can find a supportive network that acknowledges their challenges and helps them thrive in their vital roles.

7. Conclusion

Elderly care requires a holistic approach that integrates physical, emotional, and social support to meet the multifaceted needs of older adults. As individuals age, they encounter unique challenges, including chronic health conditions, cognitive decline, and social isolation. Recognizing these challenges is essential for creating a compassionate care environment that honors their dignity and enhances their overall well-being.

Comprehensive Support Systems:

To effectively support elderly individuals, it is crucial to equip both caregivers and the elderly with the appropriate tools and resources. This includes promoting awareness of health management, nutrition, and hydration, while also prioritizing mental health and emotional support. Caregivers play a pivotal role in this process; by ensuring they have access to training, respite care, and community resources, we can enhance their capacity to provide high-quality care.

Promoting Dignity and Comfort:
Additionally, fostering social engagement and facilitating community connections can significantly improve the quality of life for elderly individuals. By encouraging activities that promote social interactions and emotional well-being, we help combat loneliness and bolster mental health. Ultimately, our collective goal should be to create an environment where aging is viewed as a natural progression of life—characterized by respect, comfort, and dignity.

By acknowledging the unique needs of the elderly and implementing a comprehensive support system, we can ensure that every individual experiences the aging process as a fulfilling chapter of their life rather than a burden.

www.ingramcontent.com/pod-product-compliance
Lightning Source LLC
Chambersburg PA
CBHW040326220526
45473CB00009B/2580